SEX

FOR

DUMMIES®

Library of Congress Cataloging-in-Publication Number 99-075089

ISBN 0-7624-0750-6

This book may be ordered by mail from the publisher. Please include
$1.00 for postage and handling.
But try your bookstore first!

Running Press Book Publishers
125 South Twenty-second Street
Philadelphia, Pennsylvania 19103-4399

Visit us on the web!
www.runningpress.com

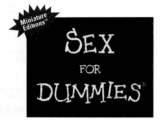

Miniature Editions

Sex

for

Dummies

**A Reference
for the Rest of Us!**™

by Dr. Ruth K. Westheimer

RUNNING PRESS
PHILADELPHIA • LONDON

Icons used in this book

 This icon points out tips to enhance sexual pleasure (so you won't have to put sticky tabs on the pages).

 This icon points to practical advice and my personal thoughts on today's sexual dilemmas.

 This icon tells you when to look before you leap to stay clear of pitfalls to your relationship.

 This icon alerts you to a useful tidbit of information.

Contents

. . . .

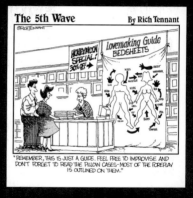

Introduction

You would think that after "doing it" for thousands of years, we all would have found a simple and effective system for passing on vital sexual information from generation to generation. But sadly, here we are, near the 21st century, and we adults continue to do a lousy job of educating ourselves and our young people about sex.

So where did most of you learn about sex? You learned a little bit from your parents and a little bit at school. But because much of this information was, rightfully, passed on before you were really ready to use it, it may not have meant all that much to you, and so it didn't totally sink in. Later on, if you had another class, you probably felt the need to act blasé, as if you knew it all, and you may not have bothered to listen.

In the end, you let trial and error become the teacher of last resort. And when that happens, not unexpectedly, you can often make serious mistakes—such as becoming pregnant when you don't intend to be, or catching a sexually transmitted disease, or, at the very least, having a less-than-satisfactory sex life, or going through your entire life never having terrific sex.

Do I encourage people to develop a relationship before they engage in sex with another person? Absolutely. And I'll say it again and again throughout this book.

But even if you're having a one-night stand that I don't approve of, I still want you to wake up the next morning healthy and safe. And I look at this book as an important tool in reaching you and others of all ages to help you discover more useful information on this important subject.

Whether you consider yourself a Don Juan, a Lady Chatterley, or a sexual novice, the first piece of advice I have for you is that everybody can become a better lover given the proper instruction. And since we

are all sexual beings,
whether we like it or not,
why not get the most out
of the pleasures our bodies
are capable of giving us? So
relax and read on. I guarantee that, by the end of this
book, you can take the dunce
cap that you may be wearing
off your head and perhaps
replace it with a condom
somewhere else!

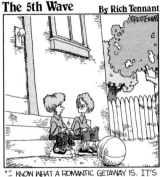

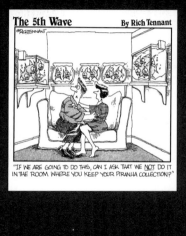

The 5th Wave   By Rich Tennant

"IF WE ARE GOING TO DO THIS, CAN I ASK THAT WE NOT DO IT IN THE ROOM WHERE YOU KEEP YOUR PIRANHA COLLECTION?"

Chapter 1

· · · · · · · · · · · · · · · · · · · ·

Getting in the Mood

*I*n its simplest form, fore-play means the touching and caressing that goes on between two people just prior to intercourse. Fore-play helps both partners experience the physical manifestations of arousal necessary for sexual satisfaction.

Foreplay for Life

According to my philosophy, not only must foreplay be

extended as long as possible when the two of you get into bed, but foreplay should begin as early as the afterplay—the caressing that goes on after sexual intercourse—of the previous sexual encounter.

In other words, I believe that afterplay can be considered part of the foreplay for the next lovemaking session, whether your next lovemaking takes place the same night or a week later.

If you're interested in becoming the best lover you can be, foreplay should be something you take into consideration with each interaction that the two of you have.

Right now, some of you are probably saying, "Hold it, Dr. Ruth, you mean to say when I ask my wife to pass the salt at dinner it's part of foreplay?"

My response is—absolutely.

Which is why you shouldn't simply say "Pass the salt," but you should add an endearment, like "Honey" or "Love" or even just her name. You see, the better you treat her, and the better she treats you, the better will be your sex life.

 If you are kind and loving even during the most mundane moments, you are setting yourself up for terrific sex when the time for lovemaking does come around.

Although I am all in favor of variety and spontaneity—so that it is quite all right to use that excitation that she is feeling and occasionally jump right into bed before going out on that date—the longer you can extend foreplay, the better the end result will usually be.

Using your lips

Kissing isn't limited to mouths. You can kiss each other all over your bodies, and both the kisser and kissee should be thoroughly enjoying the experience.

The art of massage
Make the moment as sensuous as you can.

- ✔ Dim the lights or use candles.
- ✔ Use some massage oils.
- ✔ Whatever you do, don't

rush the massage; try to really feel each other as much as possible.

✔ Alternate between strong rubs and gentle caresses. Let the sensitive nerve-endings in your fingertips help you get to know your partner in a new way.

Body mapping

Although you certainly touch your partner's body all over

during massage, the goal
then is to create sensations,
not discover which parts of
your partner's body are the
most sensitive. With body
mapping, on the other hand,
you aim to discover all of
the most sensitive parts of
one another's bodies: the
breasts, the wrists, the
thighs. . . .

Body mapping is one of
those gifts that keep on giving because, after you and

your partner have explored your bodies and discovered the most sensuous places and what feels best on them, you'll be able to use those techniques again and again throughout your love life. So body mapping is far from just a way to extend foreplay; it is an exercise that each couple should engage in at least once in order to build a data-bank of information for future lovemaking.

You have now entered . . . the erogenous zone

 Erogenous zones are the parts of your body that, due to the concentration of nerve endings, are more sensitive to stimulation than the other parts.

Now some erogenous zones are pretty universal. Most women enjoy having a man pay attention to their breasts—and most men

don't mind obliging them
in this. But, guys, don't forget what you learned in
body mapping. If she likes
a soft touch rather than a
rough one, or vice versa,
then that's what you
should do.

Remember that, in fore-
play, you're trying to arouse
each other, so you have to
do what is going to help your
partner become the most
aroused. That's not to say

that, if you really enjoy kissing her nipples but that's not number one on her list, you can't do some nipple kissing. You can, and you should. But if she really likes to have her nipples softly feathered with the tip of your finger, then you should also do some of that as well.

Erogenous zones can be anywhere on your body, but here are some of the more popular ones:

- ✔ The buttocks.
- ✔ The perineum (that little line between the anus and the genitals).
- ✔ Behind the knees.
- ✔ The nape of the neck.
- ✔ And, of course, the genitals.

Following the map

It doesn't do you any good to have a map if you don't use it, so once you've discovered which parts of the body your lover likes to have caressed,

kissed, licked, sucked, nibbled,
tickled, massaged, kneaded,
stroked, nuzzled, probed,
cupped, pinched, rubbed,
oiled, and in case I left anything out, everything else, go
ahead and do exactly that.

Switching Gears: Engaging the Genitals

No matter how long you
extend the more languorous,
romantic aspects of foreplay,

eventually you reach the point of engaging in traditional foreplay involving the genitals. Remember that the ultimate goal of foreplay is to get both partners ready to have an orgasm.

Also keep in mind that a young man does not need very much preparation, but a woman almost always does. The reasons are both physical and psychological.

Looking under the hood— foreplay for her

Most women need direct physical contact on their clitorises to have an orgasm. For the average woman, sexual intercourse alone does not give the clitoris sufficient stimulation for her to have an orgasm. This is because the penis does not come into direct contact with the clitoris during sex. One way to solve this problem is for the man to stimulate the woman's clitoris before sexual intercourse, and that is a primary function of foreplay.

In dealing with the clitoris, there is a small Catch-22. The clitoris is very sensitive, which is why it can produce an orgasm when stimulated. But, because it is so sensitive, stimulating the clitoris can also be painful. The solution to this problem is good communication between the man and the woman—and a soft touch.

 Every woman's clitoris is different, and only she knows what kind of stimulation she likes.

The tongue seems to have been perfectly constructed for the art of foreplay, and not just for kissing.

✔ Tongues provide their own lubrication in the form of saliva.

- ✔ Tongues are softer than fingertips and have no sharp instruments attached to them like nails.
- ✔ Tongues can also be manipulated in many different types of strokes, from the long lap to the short dart.

It's no wonder that a man who has per- fected the art of

cunnilingus, oral sex upon
a woman, is considered to
be a great lover by many
women.

Checking the dipstick—foreplay for him

Oral sex on a man, called
fellatio, can be performed to
various degrees. One thing
that the woman should know
is that the most sensitive
area of the penis is usually
on the underside, just below

the head, so there is no need to "deep throat" a man to give him intense pleasure.

The penis isn't the only part of the man that can be used to arouse him. Here are a few, but not all, of the parts of a man's body which can also be integrated into foreplay:

- The testicles definitely are an erogenous zone (though one that should

be handled rather gently,
because the wrong move
could put a quick end to
all the work you've put
into foreplay).

✔ Many men enjoy having
their nipples either
stroked or sucked.

✔ Also on this list of erogenous zones is the anus.
Again, be careful not to
spread germs from the
anus to other parts of
the genitals.

When to End Foreplay

How can you tell when you've had enough foreplay? You can't. Again, that's why communication is so vital to good sex. There's no right or wrong answer here. The couple should concentrate on what works best so that, in the end, both partners are satisfied. Every couple is different and so it's up to each couple to write their own ending.

As long as both partners are working towards the same goal, then the good guys (and that means both of you) will always win.

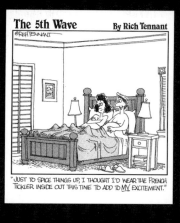

Chapter 2

. . . .

Doing It

So whether we call it "doing it," "going all the way," "having sex," or "playing hide the salami," basically we will be discussing different ways two people can help each other to experience one or more orgasms.

Although orgasm is certainly one of the goals of intercourse for both partners, how you reach that goal is where the fun comes in.

Now this is not the Kama
Sutra, so I am not going to
give you every possible
position, especially because
I don't suppose that many
of you are acrobats.

The Good Old Missionary Position

The missionary position
is no more than the male-
superior position; that is,
the man on top, woman on

the bottom, and peanut butter in between. (Scratch that last part. You'd end up sticking to each other and have to call 911.)

The missionary position is not entirely static, as there are variations. Although the woman has to spread her legs to allow the man entry, she doesn't just have to lie flat on her back. Most women bend their knees somewhat, but they can actually put their knees in a whole range of positions, including wrapped around the man's back.

In the missionary position, the man doesn't have quite the same range of motion that the woman has, but he can try to ride higher—that is, in a more upright position—which may allow his pubic bone to rub against the clitoris, giving it more stimulation.

A variation of the missionary position is to have the woman lie back on the edge of the bed or table or boat deck (see, I never want you to become predictable) while the man keeps his feet on the ground, assuming this platform is the right height to allow penetration comfortably for both. Because his weight is no longer on his arms, the man can now use his hands to touch the woman's clitoris and stimulate her to orgasm.

The Female-Superior Position

Now that we are approaching equality of the sexes, there's no reason for only men to take the superior position. We do know that more women are going on top of their men than did a decade or two ago.

It's kind of surprising that the female-superior position isn't more popular, actually, because the female-superior position offers several major advantages:

- ✔ The most important advantage of the female-superior position is that the man can caress the woman's clitoris with his fingers.
- ✔ The man can both see and fondle the woman's

breasts—a double turn-on
for men, who are more
visually oriented when it
comes to sex.

✔ Men also report being
able to "last" longer in the
female-superior position.

✔ From the woman's point
of view, she can control
the depth of penetration
and speed of thrust
(which sound more like
the controls on a Boeing
747 than sexual descrip-

tions). Because every woman develops her own unique pattern that suits her best, this kind of control can be very helpful to bring her to a fulfilling orgasm.

The female-superior position can be more tiring to the woman, especially if it takes her a while to have her orgasm. But, although some women find being on top a bit too athletic for their enjoyment, it's a position worth attempting at least once in a while.

In case you're assuming that the woman always has to be facing the man's head when she goes on top, that is not the case. She can also turn around so that her buttocks are facing his face. In fact, in the same love-making session she can turn both ways (or spin like a top, if she's so inclined).

Taking Her from Behind

The taking-her-from-behind position is not anal sex but vaginal sex, where the man enters the woman from behind, the way most animals do. Penetration can be a little more tricky to achieve this way, but most couples can figure out a way to make this position work for them.

Doggy style, as this position is called, allows the man

to reach around and stimulate the woman's clitoris and also gives him an exciting rear view that many men like. This position can be a little hard on the woman's knees, but that is basically its only drawback. One reason this position is not more popular is probably that the woman's view isn't very scenic, unless there's a nice Cezanne landscape in front of her, or a mirror.

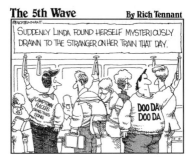

The standing canine

Depending on the height of the two partners, rear entry can sometimes be accomplished while both partners have their feet on the ground, with the woman bending over, probably holding onto a chair or some other sturdy object.

This is one of those semi-acrobatic positions that are good for adding variety and keeping boredom out of the bedroom, but not always satisfactory to either partner because the couple has to concentrate on their sexual arousal while also trying to keep their balance.

Splitting the difference

Another position, called the cuissade, is half-missionary and half-rear-entry (and maybe half-baked, too, but I don't want any of you to accuse me of having left out your favorite position).

✔ The woman lies on her back but turns half way and puts her leg up into the air (she gets extra points from the judges if she keeps her toes pointed North).

✔ The man straddles the leg on the bed and enters her, while holding himself up with his arms.

This position will definitely cause some heavy breathing, but whether or not any orgasms result will depend mostly on your physical stamina.

Spooning

Another variation of the doggy style, and a much more relaxing one, is the spoon position. Here, the man still enters the woman's vagina from the back but, instead of the woman being on her knees, she's lying down on her side. Many cou-

ples are familiar with this
position because it's only a
short thrust away from a
position in which they sometimes sleep.

East Side, West Side, Side by Side

In the side-by-side position,
also called the scissors position, the woman lies on her
back and the man lies next
to her; he swivels his hips,

interlaces his legs with hers, and enters her vagina from the side. If you're not very good at tying knots, then you may have some initial difficulties getting into this position, but it is a very good one, so don't give up. (If you really have difficulties, contact your nearest sailor.)

Here, again, the man can easily stimulate the woman's clitoris

while thrusting inside of her,
as well as touch her breasts
(and she can touch his).
Each partner can see the
other's face and, if the tem-
perature is low (or modesty
is high), everyone can stay
snugly under the covers.
It makes you wonder why
you'd even bother with the
missionary position (unless
you have some missionaries
visiting you from the South
Pacific).

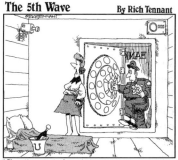

The 5th Wave

By Rich Tennant

"Oh, wait a minute Arthur! When I said I'd only have safe sex with you, this isn't what I meant!"

Lap Dancing

The basic idea, when not done
in public, is for the man to sit
down and the woman to then
sit on top of him so that his
penis slips into her vagina.
If the woman is sitting so
that she is facing him, she
doesn't have the control over
thrusting that she does in the
female-superior position, and,
with a woman sitting on top
of him, the man can't do very

much thrusting either. But, if you sit on his penis with your back to him, then you can keep your feet on the floor and go up and down as you would in the female-superior position.

The Oceanic Position

What positions did the natives in the South Pacific favor before those missionaries got there? One, which has

been nicknamed the Oceanic
Position, would be just about
impossible for most Western-
ers of today. It seems that,
because the natives didn't
have chairs, they spent a lot
time squatting, which they
then adapted to sex. The
woman lies down and
spreads her legs and the
man then squats over her
and inserts his penis into her.
Supposedly, this gave the
man the ability to prolong

intercourse for long periods. But, unless they happen to be catchers on a baseball team, I doubt that most men could last very long at all in this position.

Standing Up

Unless your bodies match up perfectly well in terms of height and shape, the standing-up position winds up being a difficult one to

achieve. If the man is strong
enough, he can pick the
woman up so that they can
fit, but the exertion is likely
to lessen his enjoyment, to
say the least.

The standing-up position
is sometimes depicted with
both partners in the shower.
It appears to be very romantic, but more accidents occur
in the bath and shower than
anywhere else, including our
nation's highways.

I am all for experimentation and making sex fun, but sex isn't an athletic event. Nor are any Olympic medals given out for degrees of sexual difficulty. Orgasms by themselves are a great reward, and, if you can have them without risking life and limb, then I see no reason to go the extreme route. On the other hand, while I like to ski down a mountain, other

people like to hot-dog it, so if
you can experiment safely,
and it gives you an extra
kick, be my guest.

Oral Sex: Using Your Mouth

One area I haven't touched
upon yet are the positions
that you can use for oral sex.
Certainly there is no right
way or wrong way; whatever
suits you is best. But one

way does have a name of its own—"69," which refers to mutual oral sex. The name comes from the shape of two bodies as they lie against each other, upside down to one another. Although it really doesn't matter which partner is on top, the man usually is the one to assume this role because he is likely to have to strain his neck more if he is on the bottom. (Sometimes a pillow under his neck can help.) It may be most comfortable for both partners if both lie on their sides.

The Big O

Unfortunately, some people adopt a take-it-or-leave-it attitude towards orgasms. But, without orgasms, probably none of us would be here. After all, it's because men and women seek this

intense instant of pleasure
that people have managed
to hang onto this planet by
reproducing themselves over
the millennia. So we have a
lot to be thankful for when
it comes to orgasms, and
we shouldn't take them
for granted.

What is an orgasm, anyway?

An orgasm is an intense feeling of physical pleasure that
we human beings experience

as the culmination of sexual stimulation. When you experience an orgasm, your breathing becomes fast and heavy, your pulse races, the deep muscles in the genital area contract, and your toes may even curl up. In men, orgasm is almost always accompanied by ejaculation, the forceful ejection of semen from the penis, necessary for procreation. Women also feel orgasms, although their orgasms are not needed for procreation.

Climaxing during Intercourse

Having sex with someone is not like being a trapeze artist, where the timing has to be just right or else one of you falls to the ground. If you can have simultaneous orgasms, even once in a while, great, but don't make a big deal out of it if you can't. You're more likely to ruin your sex lives than to perfect them.

Multiple orgasms

Are two orgasms better than one? How about three, four, five, or six? Only the individual can answer that question.

Although all orgasms are pleasurable, they are not all identical.

The G-spot myth or fact?

Forty years ago, a gynecologist named Ernest Grafenberg claimed to have found a spot in the vagina that seemingly could give women orgasms without clitoral stimulation. In 1982, three researchers wrote a book about this spot, calling it the Grafenberg Spot, or G-spot, and ever since its publication, I am constantly being asked questions by women desperately looking for their own G-spots. One reason these women are so concerned is that a G-spot orgasm is supposed to be much stronger than a mere clitoral orgasm; it may even include a supposed female ejaculation.

It seems odd to me that such a wonderful thing as the G-spot wasn't better known before recently. I've spoken to many gynecologists, and none has been able to provide me with any hard evidence of its existence. More research has been done, but I haven't seen anything to convince me that this G-spot definitely exists.

Now I'm not against the G-spot. After all, if there is some special place within the vagina that gives women fabulous orgasms, who am I to complain? My problem with the G-spot is that there has never been any scientifi-

cally validated proof that
it exists. Yet thousands, and
for all I know, millions of
women are now looking for
their G-spots.

Actually, because of where
the G-spot is said to be located,
a woman would have a very
hard time finding it by herself.
Instead, she has to send her
partner on a Lewis and Clark
expedition up her vagina.
When they don't find this pot
of gold, some women blame

their men for being inadequate explorers. Then the two of them end up having a fight over it, and their entire sex life goes down the tubes.

I'm not a big believer in lotteries, but every once in a while, when the jackpot gets really big, I go out and spend a couple of bucks on a ticket. The odds are long, but so what, how much have I wasted? That's my philosophy

about the G-spot. If a couple
wants to look for the
woman's G-spot, it's no big
deal, as long as they don't
invest too much in this
search. If they find a place
in her vagina that gives her
a lot of pleasure, great. If
they don't, they should just
forget about it.

Don't try—let it come
When it comes to sex, we
humans cannot be too aware

of what we are doing or our sexual powers go haywire. Anytime we become overly conscious of the sexual process, we begin to lose our ability to perform. This is particularly true for men who have difficulties having an erection. If they enter a sexual situation expecting to fail, it's almost guaranteed that they will. The same can be true for a woman who has any difficulties attaining an orgasm. If she is trying too hard to climax, it will only make it more difficult for her to do so.

If you're lucky, an experience like the simultaneous orgasm will happen by itself once in a while and provide some extra enjoyment. But if you try too hard, the odds are against it happening at all.

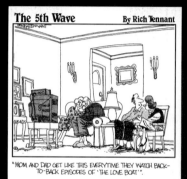

The 5th Wave

By Rich Tennant

"MOM AND DAD GET LIKE THIS EVERYTIME THEY WATCH BACK-TO-BACK EPISODES OF 'THE LOVE BOAT'."

Chapter 3

· · · · · · · · · · · · · · · · · · · ·

Keeping the
Fires Burning

*I*f you want to become a terrific lover, especially in showing your partner that you really love her, then knowledge of afterplay is vital. So I want you to pay close attention.

The Simplest of Techniques

In terms of technique, there's not really all that much to afterplay. We're not talking rocket science here. In fact, we're not even talking paper airplane making.

All afterplay requires is that the man take a little bit of time to hold and caress his partner, both physically and verbally, after she has had her orgasm. Does that sound complicated? Or strenuous? Should it tax the intelligence or the stamina of either the strongest or weakest of men? Of course not.

Afterplay creates foreplay

Men who take time for afterplay will be rewarded not
only with more satisfied,
and hence happier, wives or
lovers, but also with better
sex lives. You see, I look at
afterplay as really the begin-
ning of foreplay for the next
sexual episode. The more
you stretch out foreplay, the
better sex will be the next
time. So if you can start foreplay with afterplay right after

you have sex, you won't be wasting a single second. Just imagine what that's going to do for your sex life!

Use Variety to Spice Up Your Sex Life

Variety adds to romance in many ways. If you always go to the same restaurant when you go out to dinner, that can get boring, and boredom doesn't help keep those

romantic fires burning. The
need for variety is also true
in the bedroom.

 If you always make
love exactly the
same way, it can
become boring.

Make some new moves

I'm not saying you have to go
to Fantasy Island every time
you make love. Even if you
make love the same way nine
out of ten times, at least that

tenth time, try something a
little different. If you stay in
the same rut, it will only get
more and more entrenched,
and then you'll never be able
to get out of it.

Variety can mean making
love someplace you've never
done it, like the kitchen floor
or on the dining-room table
(just make sure that the legs
are darn sturdy). You can
add variety by making love
at a different time of the day,

like early in the morning or
in the middle of the after-
noon. You can make love
with most of your clothes
on—or with only one of you
naked and the other one fully
clothed. Let your imagina-
tion fly and see where it
takes you.

 The one thing I must
caution you about,
however, is never to
pressure your partner into
doing something that he or

she doesn't want to do. It's
fine to be creative, but you
have to create something
you'll both enjoy.

Don't be a lazy lover

You know that you only get
negative results from being
lazy at school or at work, so
why do you think that you
can be lazy when it comes to
sex? A lazy lover is a lousy
lover. The more energy you
put into your lovemaking,

the better a lover you'll be.

Now, by energy, I don't necessarily mean more physical energy, although that's worth trying if the two of you tend to be passive. The energy I'm talking about is spirit. The more of yourself you put into your love making, the more you'll get out of it.

Take charge of your sex life, and you can achieve tremendous results.

Create an adventure

In addition to using variety, it's also important to be a little daring. Take a risk on a new position. What's the worst that can happen? Now when I say don't be afraid to take risks, I'm not suggesting you do anything really dangerous, especially concerning unsafe sex. But, within reason, the sex act has many variations that don't involve any real harm beyond the risk that one or both of you won't be able to sustain the position or have an orgasm. So you miss one orgasm, that's no big deal. On the other hand, if you decide that you like a new position, it can bring you many, many orgasms over the course of a lifetime.

Visit a sex shop

Many people wouldn't be caught dead in a sex shop,

and my question to them is:
Why not? When you're
hungry, you go to the super-
market. When you need
clothes, you go to a
department store.

So, if you need a
little more variety
in your sex life,
what's wrong with going to
a sex shop?

What might you find in one
of these stores? There are
many different varieties of sex

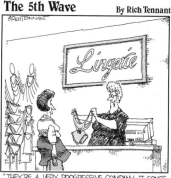

The 5th Wave
By Rich Tennant

"THEY'RE A VERY PROGRESSIVE COMPANY—IT COMES WITH MATCHING COLORED CONDOMS."

stores. Some feature mostly
X-rated movies. Others have
a large selection of so-called
marital aids, like vibrators
and dildos. Some have sexy
lingerie, while others have
lots of leather products. Sex
stores often cater to a partic-
ular audience, so that one
store may have a lot of whips
and chains, and another
won't have any.

Whatever you do, don't
go into a sex store with a

serious attitude, or you'll wind up being disappointed. Sex is supposed to be fun, and the gadgets and gizmos featured in these stores are supposed to add to the fun of lovemaking. If you're not comfortable using any of these products, then simply browse.

Use a mail-order catalog

If you don't dare go into a sex store, or if there's not

one near you, the next best thing is to get a catalog. That way, you can do your browsing without fear of the neighbors peeking in. All adult catalog companies send their catalogs in plain wrappers, and the same goes when they ship their merchandise, so even your mail carrier won't suspect a thing.

There are different catalogs for different tastes.

Watch X-rated videos

Although there are certainly X- or NC-17-rated movies in America that I would object to, in general, I am in favor of people renting erotic films. For couples, viewing such films can provide both some added spice and maybe even the knowledge of some new positions or techniques to their sexual repertoire. European films are much more sophisticated

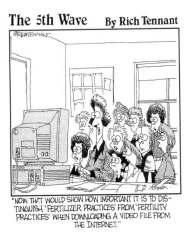

"NOW THAT WOULD SHOW HOW IMPORTANT IT IS TO DISTINGUISH 'FERTILIZER PRACTICES' FROM 'FERTILITY PRACTICES' WHEN DOWNLOADING A VIDEO FILE FROM THE INTERNET."

in this respect, providing truly artistic treatment of sexual subjects.

I just called to say . . .

The phone can be a helpful tool to spice up your sex life, even if you're married. When you talk on the phone, you're speaking right into the other person's ear. Whispering "sweet nothings"—or "hot somethings"—into the phone, so that only your

lover and you can hear
them, can let you get up
close and personal at any
time of the day or night. You
can use these moments as
part of your overall strategy
for foreplay.

 And, if the circum-
stances are right,
once in a while you
can even have real phone
sex, with one or both of you
masturbating, just to throw
in some variety.

Fantasy

There's no such thing as a wrong fantasy. In fantasy, you don't have to worry about safer sex, what the neighbors would say, or anything else. If you want to make love to Alexander the Great and his whole army, be my guest. If you want to fantasize about Hannibal and his elephants, go ahead. Literally, whatever turns you on is A-OK.

A question I often get asked is: "Should I share my fantasies with my spouse or lover?" The significant word here is caution. Some partners don't mind hearing their lovers' fantasies; some even get aroused by them, but some get very jealous. If you feel the need to talk about your fantasies with your partner, do it very carefully. Here are some tips:

✔ Make the first one very tame. Maybe your favorite fantasy is being a Dallas Cowboys cheerleader caught naked in the locker room with the whole team. That's fine, but tell him that it's being found naked in your office after hours by him. If he reacts positively, then you can work your way up to telling him your real fantasies down the road.

✔ Use common sense. If your husband is built like Woody Allen and you tell him you're always fantasizing about Arnold Schwarzenegger, how do you think that's going to make him feel?

✔ Remember the Golden Rule. If you tell your partner about your fantasies, be prepared to hear his or her fantasies back. If you think that you might get jealous, then don't open that Pandora's box in the first place.

My last piece of advice regarding fantasies holds true for nonsexual fantasies as well as the sexual ones, and that's to remember that they are fantasies. Fantasies are wonderful tools; just be careful how you use them.

Take Charge of Your Sex Life

The success of your sex life is not something that you should leave to chance. Work on it, and you can definitely reap rewards that are worth the effort you put in. The other side of that coin is that, if you ignore your sex life, it will be much more difficult to get those fires burning again. So take my advice and start right now.

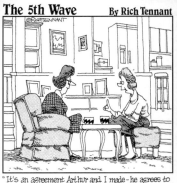

The 5th Wave   By Rich Tennant

"It's an agreement Arthur and I made - he agrees to stay home from the gym 2 nights a week, and I guarantee that he'll still burn over 300 calories each night."

Chapter 4

. . . .

Dr. Ruth's Rx
for Romance

T he key to good sexual func-
tioning is to be sexually
literate, and one important way
of earning your master's degree
in sexual literacy is to do a
little housecleaning upstairs
and sweep away any sexual
myths that have been hiding
in the corners of your brain.

Ten Dumb Things People Believe about Sex

1. If I haven't had sex by the

time I'm 18, I'm a loser.

2. The more I score, the more pleasure I'll have.

3. Being a heterosexual makes me immune to AIDS.

4. The grass is always greener in the neighbors' bedroom.

5. Having sex will make everything all right.

6. A good lover must be an open book.

7. I should always compare sexual partners.

8. I can't become a better lover.

9. Lovers are like Siamese twins.

10. I'm too old to have sex.

Ten Tips for Safer Sex

There are no absolute guarantees when it comes to having safe sex between two people, but you can enjoy safer sex if you're careful to follow the guidelines that have been developed by the experts.

1. Learn to say no.

2. Limit your number of partners.

3. Don't rely solely on your instincts.

4. Never dull your senses when you're with strangers.

5. Make the first move toward safer sex.

6. Use condoms.

7. Develop a relationship before you have sex.

8. Don't engage in risky behavior.

9. Don't forget about the other STDs.
10. Don't sell your other options short.

Ten Things Women Wish Men Knew about Sex

It's amazing to me that men are always saying that they want to have sex with women so badly but then so many of them don't put in the effort to find out what it

takes to have good sex
with a woman.

So all of you guys out there
who complain that you don't
get enough of "it," read the
following tips closely. I know
how you men often resist
asking for directions, but if
you've lost that loving feeling,
then read on with an open
mind and force yourself to
accept some guidance on
how to get to the Tunnel
of Love.

1. Chivalry isn't dead yet.
2. Appearances do count.
3. You can't hurry love.
4. A clitoris is not just a small penis.
5. Women need to bathe in the afterglow.
6. Kinky sex isn't sexy sex.
7. Wandering eyes mean less sex.
8. Slam-bam-thank-you-ma'am doesn't cut the mustard.
9. Changing diapers is sexy.

10. Just because you can't doesn't mean you won't.

Ten Things Men Wish Women Knew about Sex

Ladies, if any of you out there still believe that the way to a man's heart is through his stomach, then you have a lot to learn. Between fast food franchises, pizza, and Chinese take-out, men are quite capable of feeding themselves.

Now just because a man's apparatus is on view doesn't mean it's all that simple to operate. And while there are auto mechanics to look under the hood of your car, I don't think you want anyone else changing the oil (tinkering with the cylinders, lubricating the ball joint, lifting the valves) of your man, so pay attention to these tips if you want to get the most from your relationship.

1. Try not to give mixed signals.

2. It really does hurt.

3. Sometimes it's OK not to save electricity.

4. The Playboy playmate is not a threat.

5. Teamwork is important.

6. The day I stop looking is the day I'm dead.

7. If you really loved me you'd . . .

8. The way to a man's heart is not through his stomach.

9. To a man, sex is different than love.

10. The older a man gets, the more help he needs.

Ten Tips for Truly Great Lovers

Anybody can teach you how to make love, but I, Dr. Ruth, want you to become not just any kind of lover, but a truly great lover. I want you and your partner to have

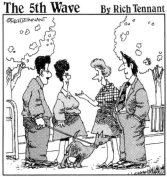

"We met on the Internet and I absolutely fell in looove with his syntax."

terrrrific sex, and to do that you have to learn how to roll your Rs and heed the following tips.

1. Don't make love on your first date.

2. Set the mood as far in advance as possible.

3. Find out what your partner needs.

4. Protect yourself and your partner.

5. Don't fall into a rut.

6. Address your problems.

7. Use your sense of touch.

8. Become a great kisser.

9. Satisfy your partner even if you don't feel like sex.

10. Learn to adapt to your circumstances.

This book has been bound
using handcraft methods and
Smyth-sewn to ensure durability.

The dust jacket and interior were
designed by Terry Peterson.

The cartoons are
by Rich Tennant.

The text was edited
by Marc Frey.

The text was set in
ITC Cheltenham and
Cascade Script.

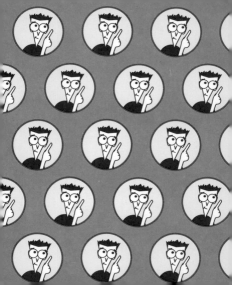